Today is an exciting day! It is Arun's 10th birthday! Arun and his family are having a small party at their home to celebrate. Andy, Arun's best friend, is invited to the party.

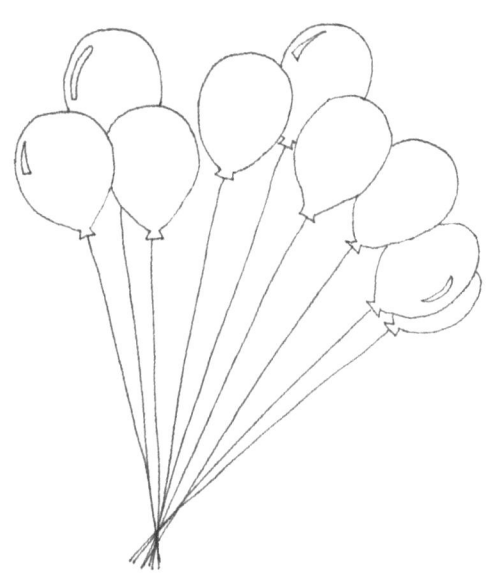

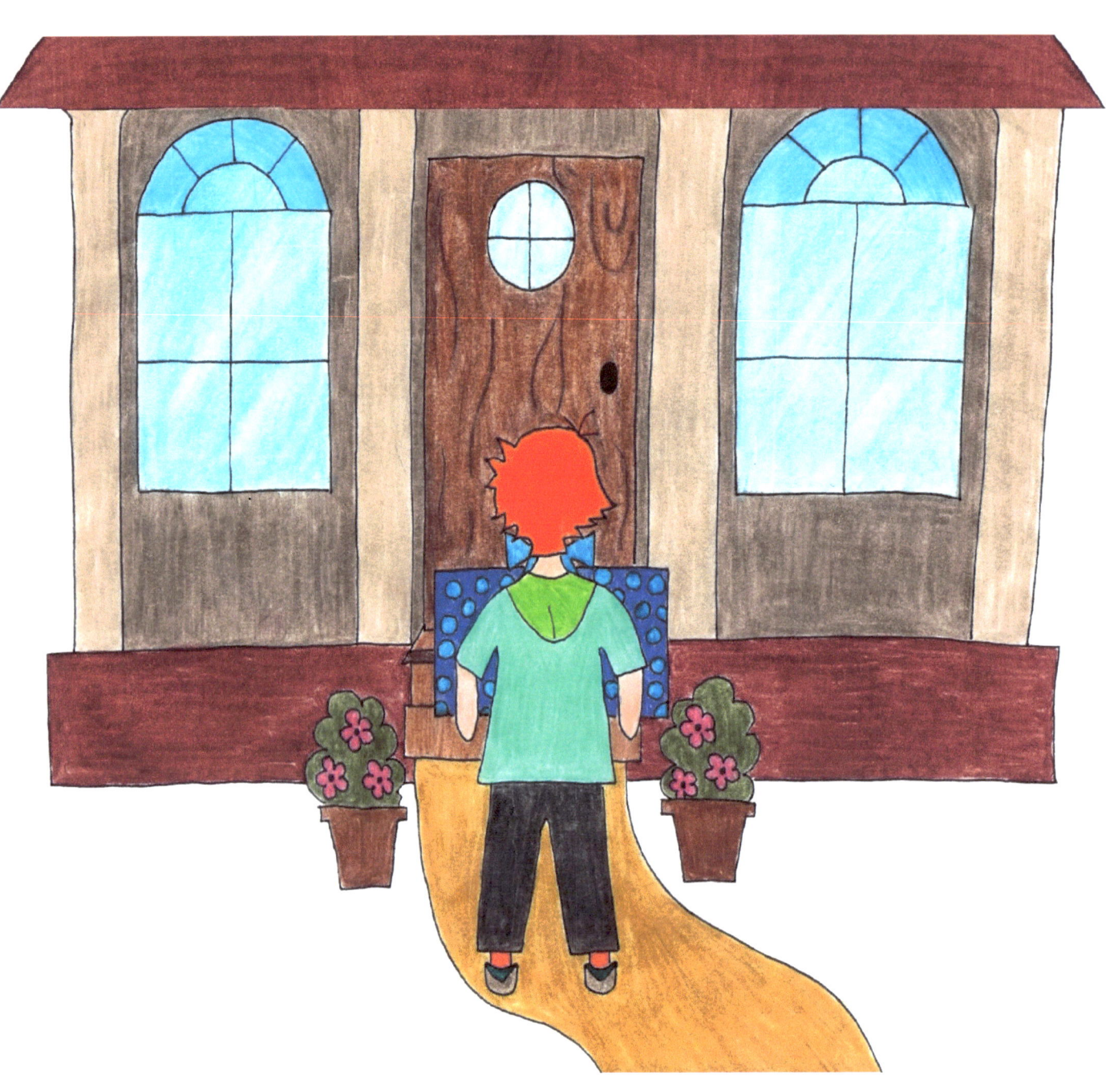

Since Arun's home is just down the street from Andy's, Andy decided he would walk. Andy got dressed and rushed out the door with a huge present to give Arun. It's something Andy knew Arun always wanted.

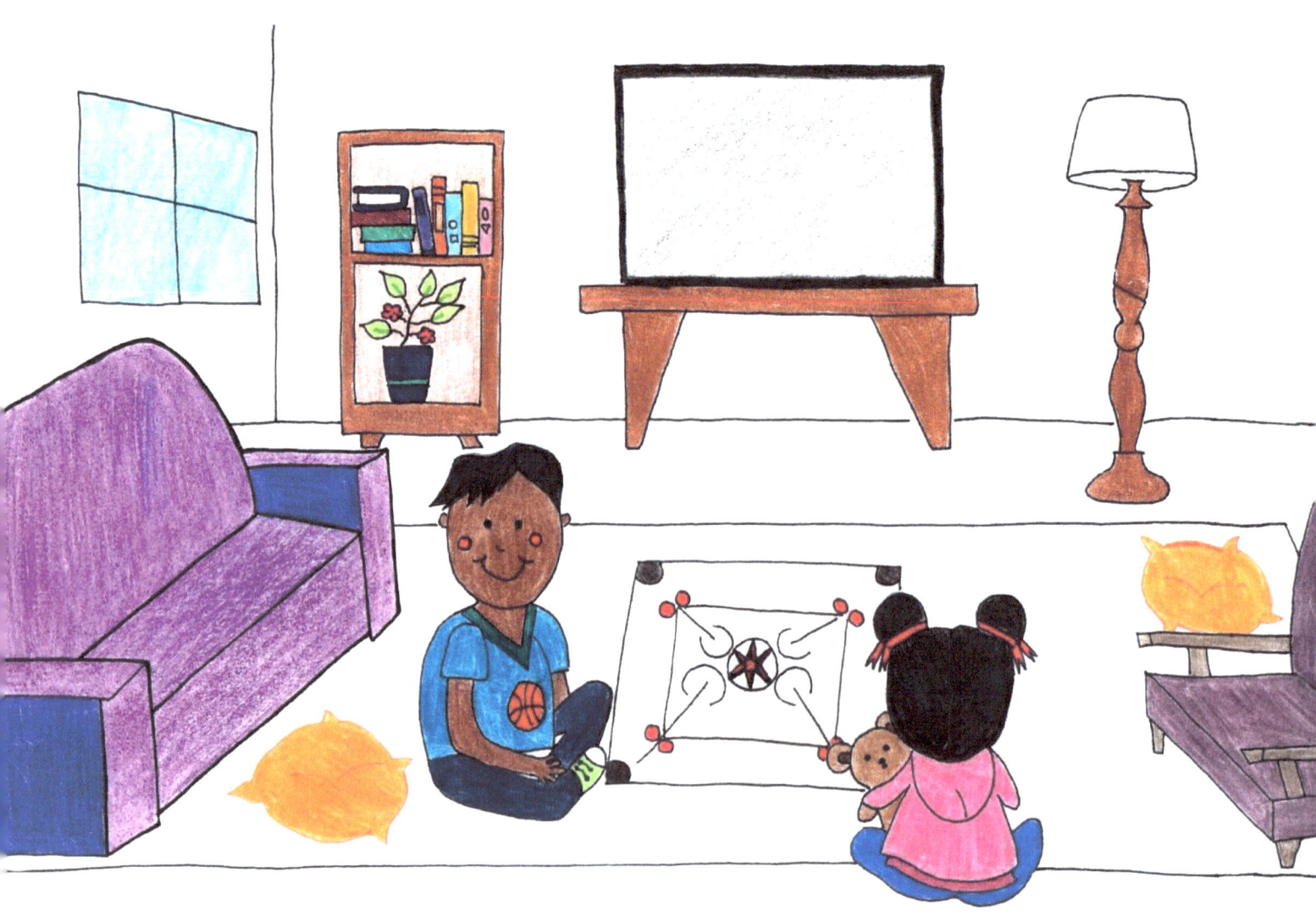

Arun, like many Indian boys, lives in a *joint family*. A joint family means Arun, his Mummy, his Papa, his younger sister Neha, and his two grandparents Dada and Dadi, from Papa's side, all live in the same home.

Together they help each other.

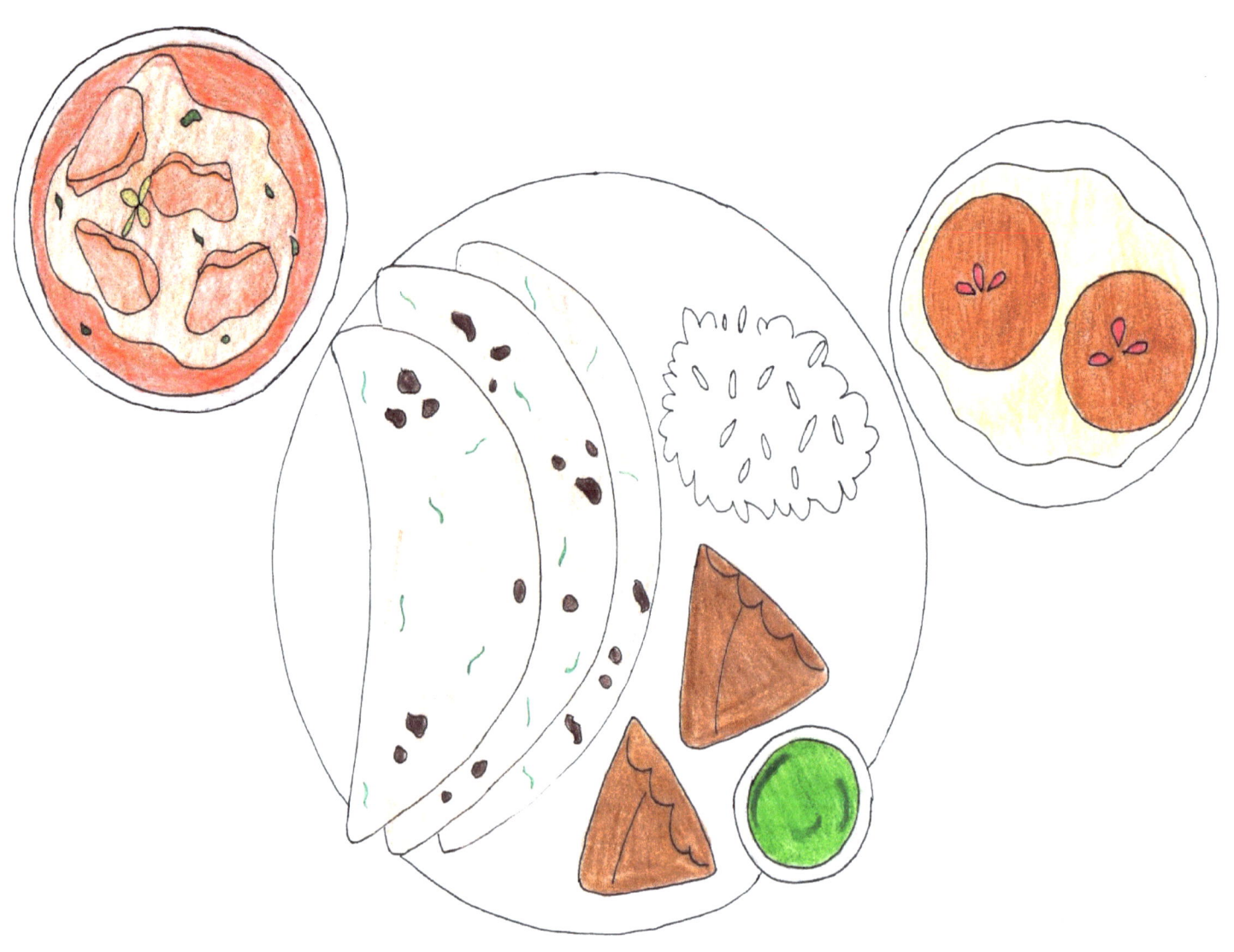

Arun's family is always excited to see Andy and they oftentimes offer Andy good food. However, today is going to be extra special because of Arun's birthday!

Arun's Mummy is cooking butter chicken, rice, naan, lots of Indian desserts, as well as cake! All of which is Arun's favorite and secretly Andy's too. Yum! Andy's mouth began to water just at the thought of it.

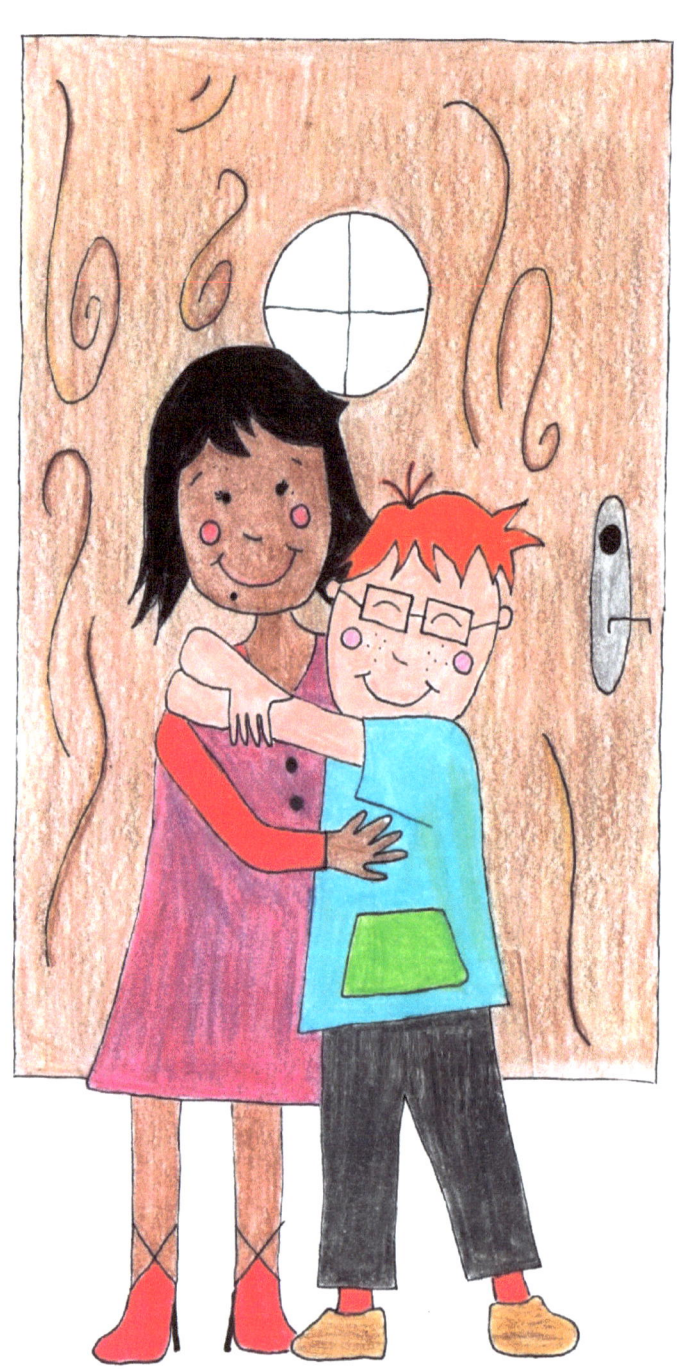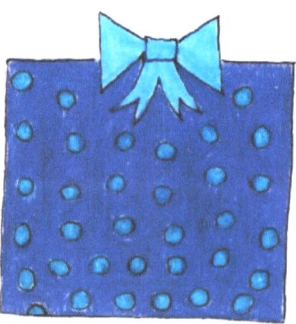

"Hi, Andy!" Arun's Mummy squeezed Andy in a blanketing-hug as she greeted him at the front door.

"Arun, your friend is here!"

she shouted to her son.

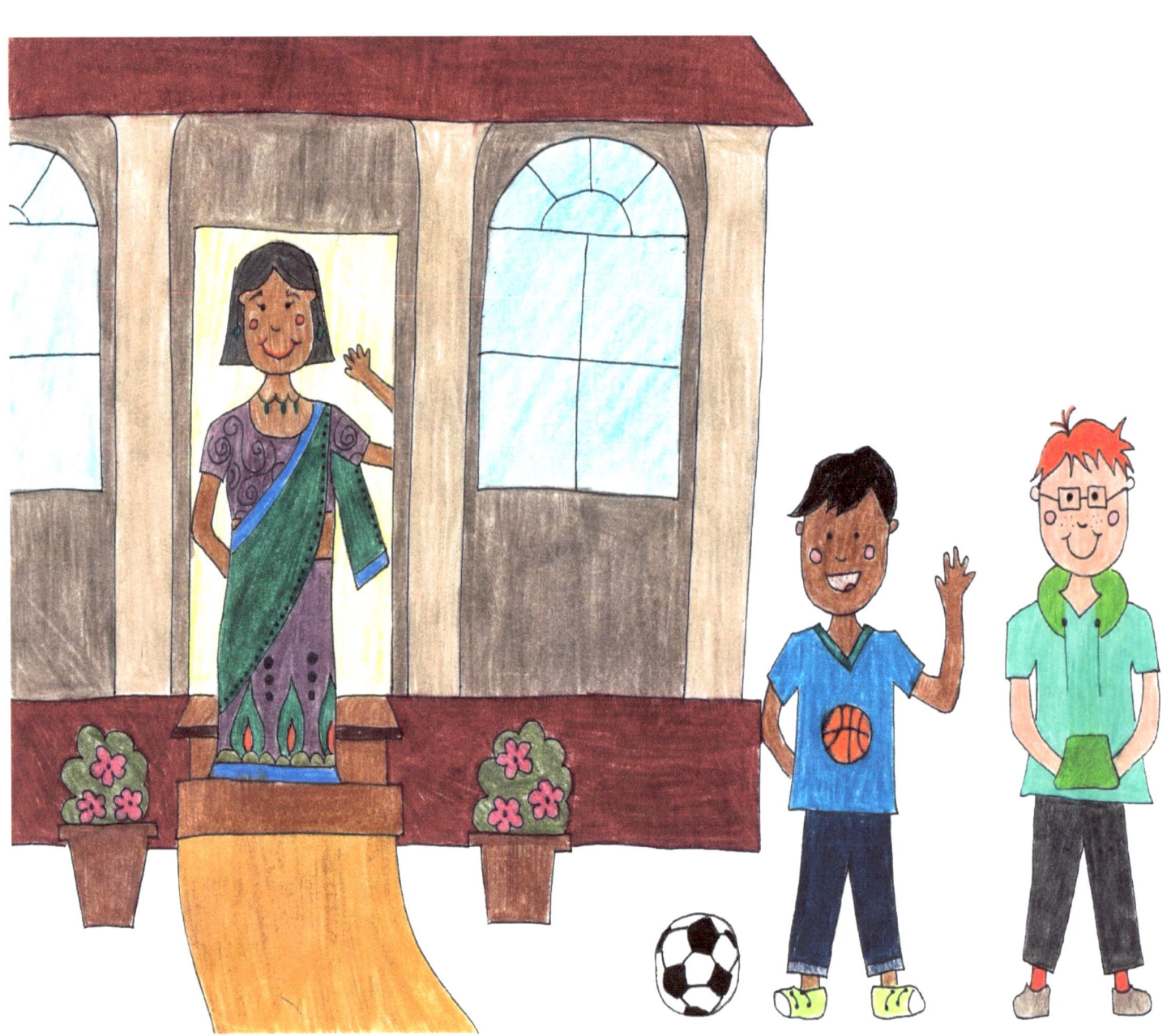

Arun ran toward Andy excitedly. He opened his birthday gift and thanked Andy.

"I love it!" exclaimed Arun.

He then grabbed Andy's hand and they both hurried outside to play.

As soon as lunch was ready Dadi, Arun's grandma, called out, "Arun beta, it's time to come inside. Bring your friend and make sure to wash your hands.

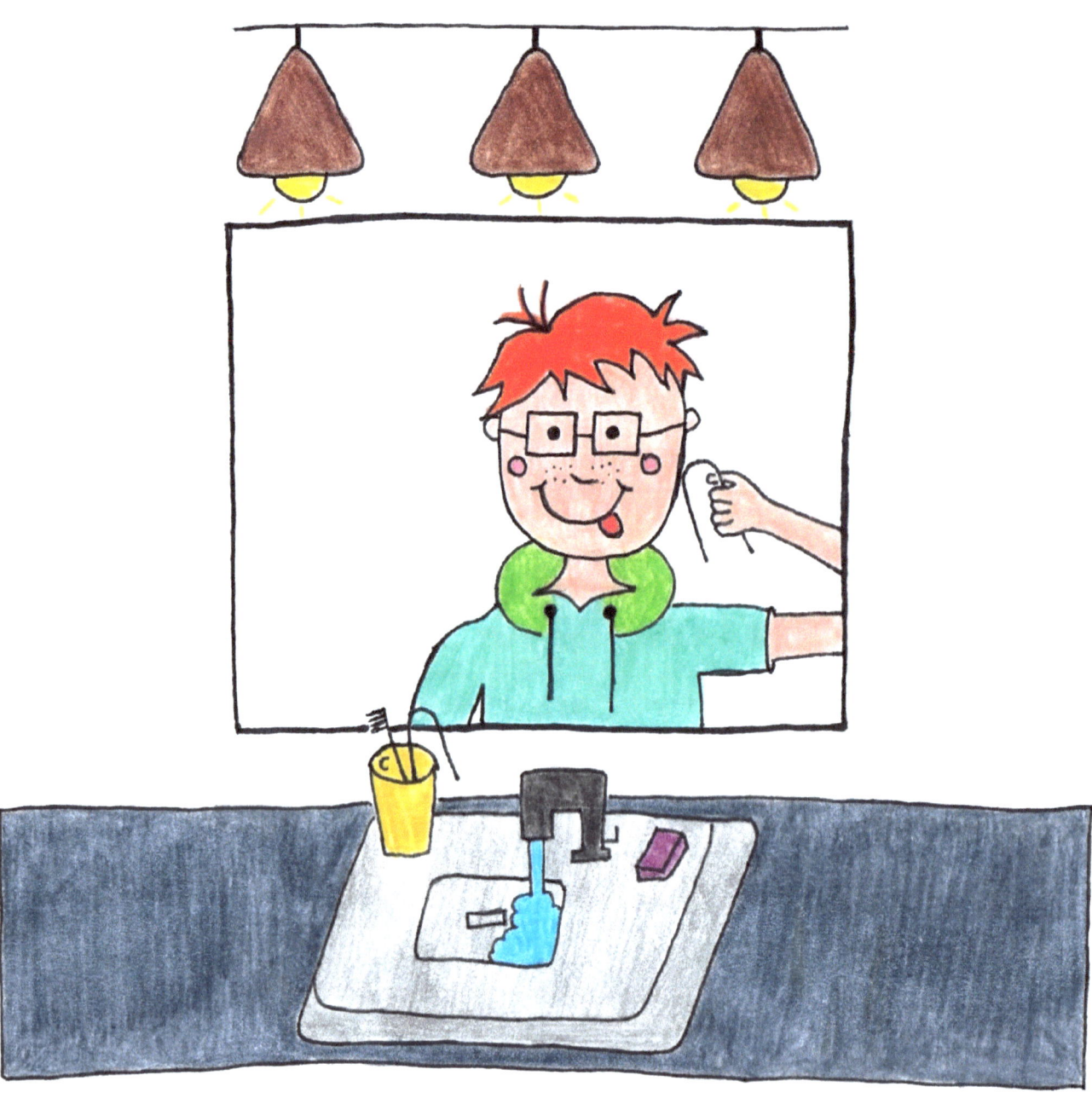

"OK, Dadi!" Arun answered. He headed toward the kitchen, while Andy rushed into the bathroom.

Meanwhile, Arun looked around to see if everything for the lunch party was ready.

While Andy was washing his hands, he noticed something different in the toothbrush holder sitting on the side of the sink.

"Hmm, that's interesting" Andy mumbled.

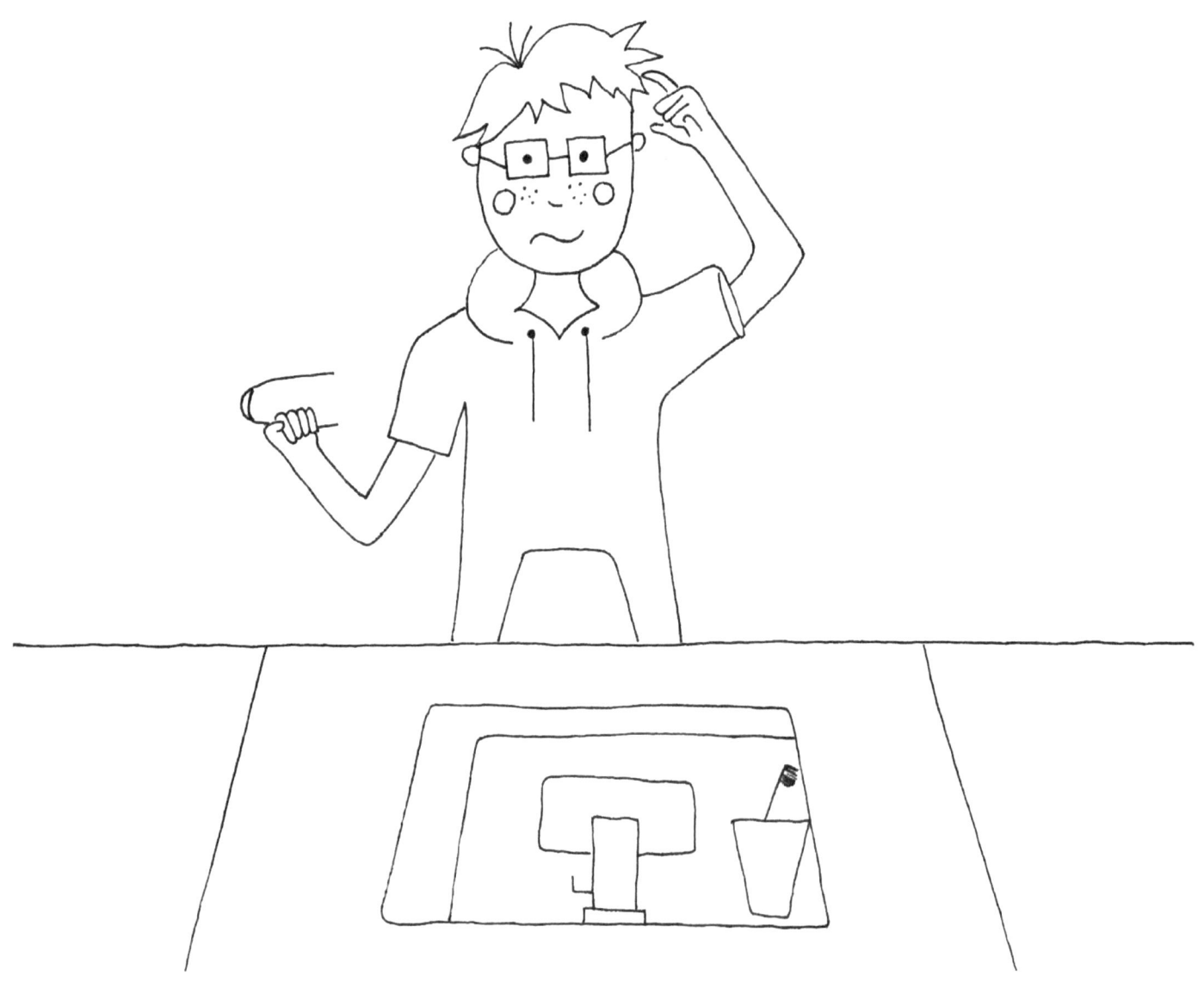

Andy noticed a metal "u-shaped" object in the holder alongside a toothbrush. He picked it up and turned it over and over wondering what it was used for.

At first, Andy felt the edges along the curve. It looked sharp, but to his surprise, it wasn't.

"This can't be a razor for shaving. I wonder what it is, then?" thought Andy.

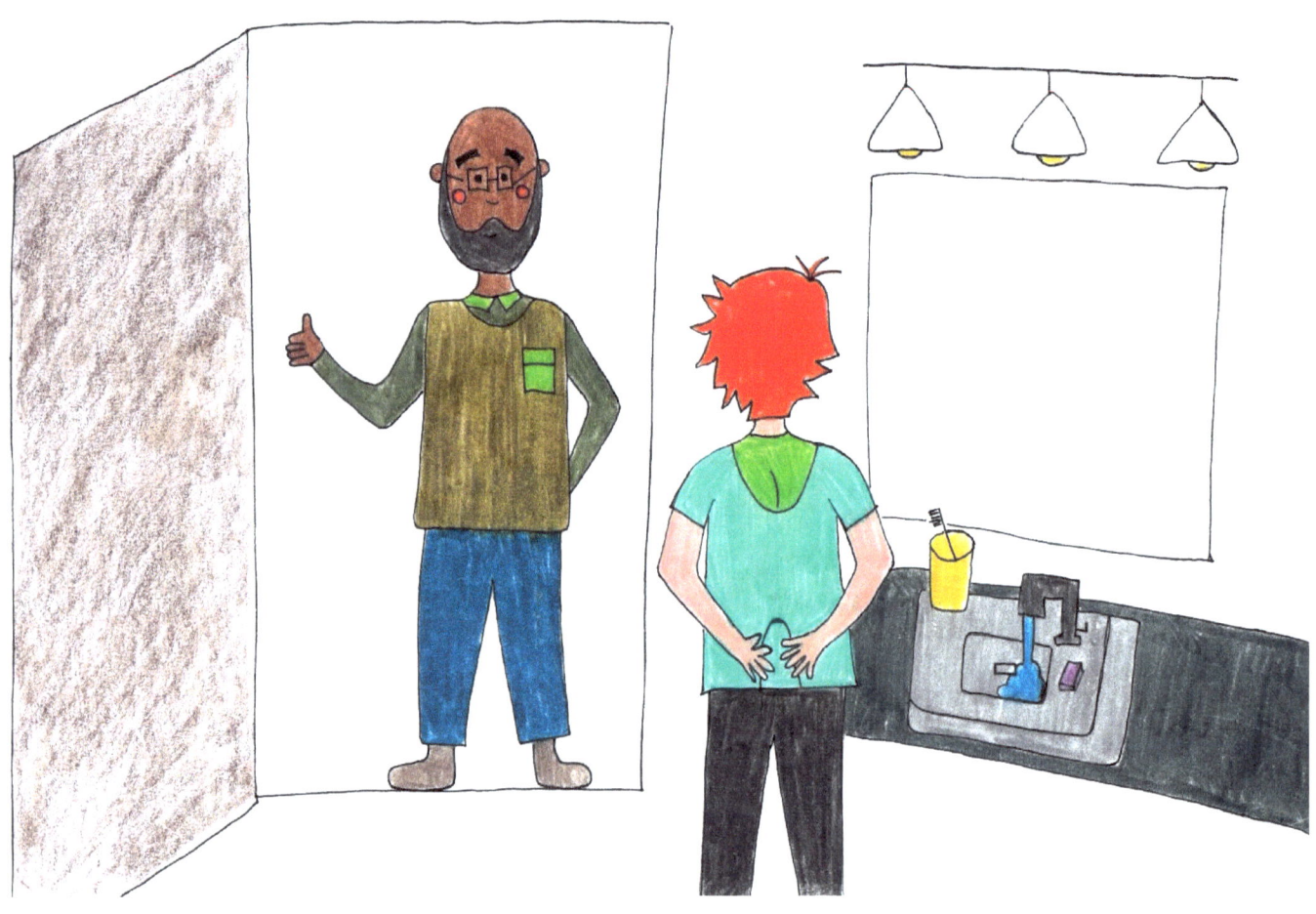

Moments later, someone knocked on the door. "Coming!" Andy shouted.

As Andy quickly opened the bathroom door, he was surprised to see Arun's grandpa, Dada, standing there! Suddenly, Andy accidentally dropped the metal piece!

"Oops! Um, uh, sorry, sir," stuttered an embarrassed Andy.

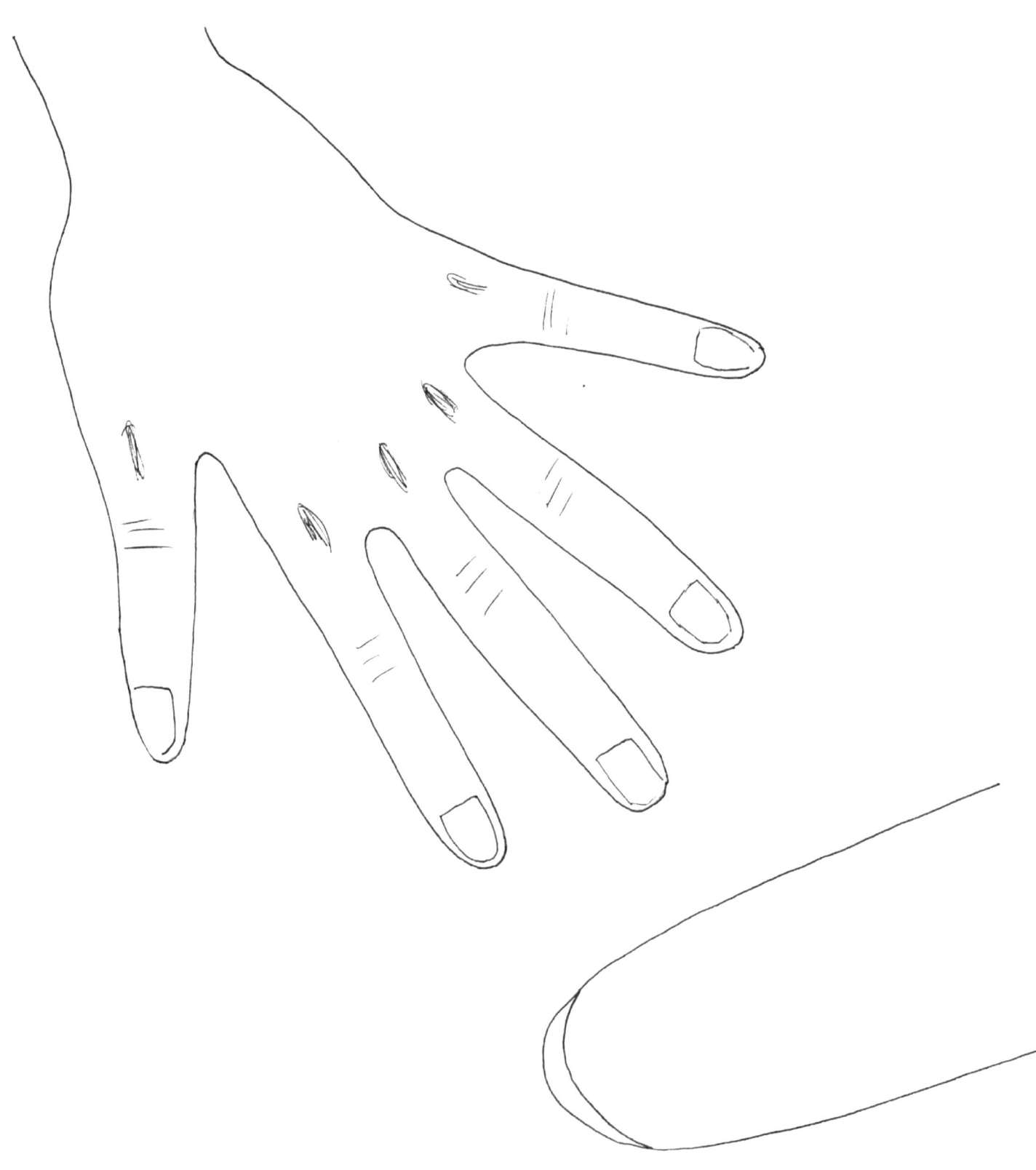

Dada's eyes went straight to the metal object that was now laying on the bathroom floor.

"Andy, did you drop this? "Dada pointed.

"Um, yes, I did, "Andy hesitated.

There was a moment of silence.

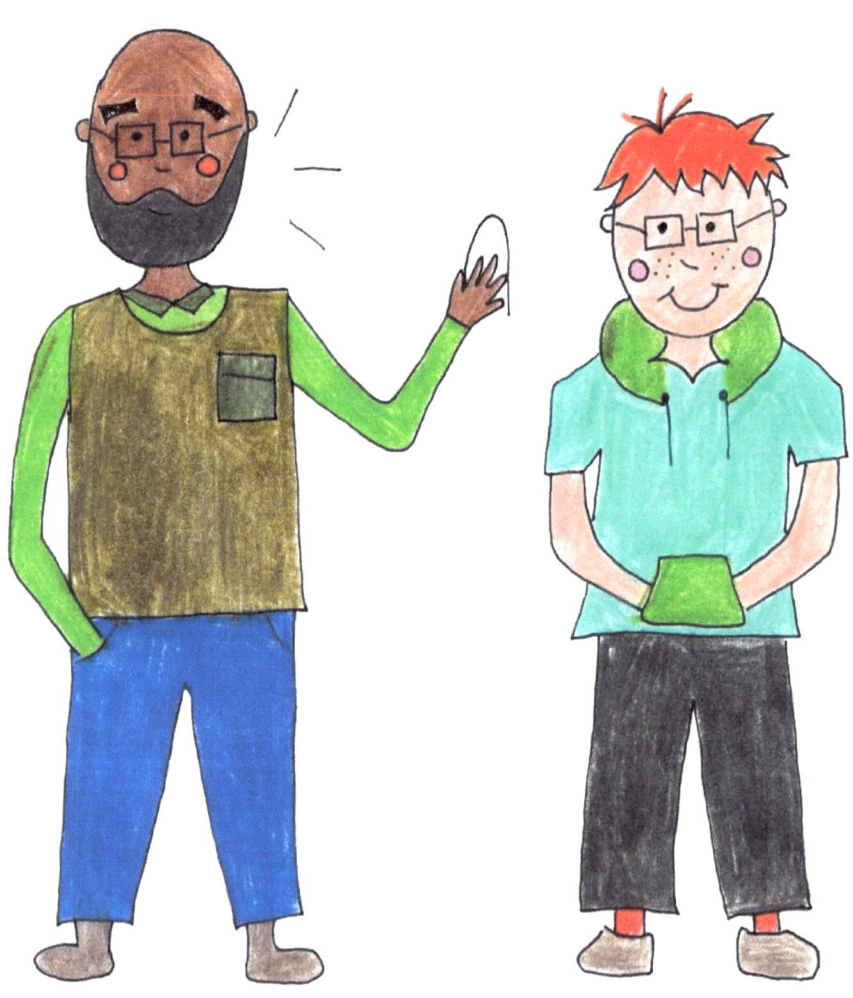

Dada cleared his throat, picked up the object and asked Andy," Do you know what this is?"

"No, sir," said Andy, "I was curious so that's why I took it out of the toothbrush holder. I accidentally dropped it. I'm sorry. It looks weird to me."

"That is okay, Andy. Let's eat lunch and I'll explain it all, "Dada said.

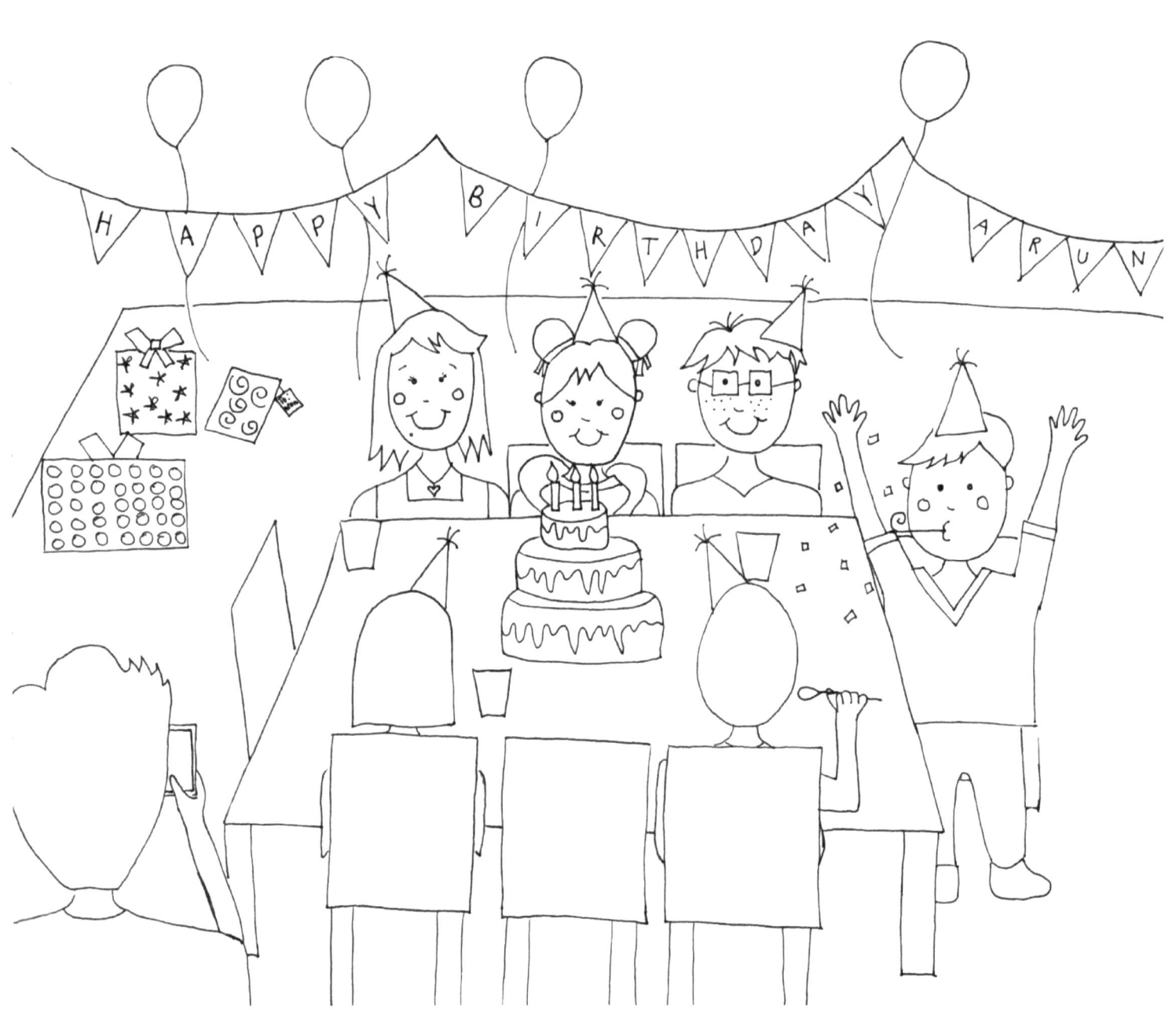

Arun's family and Andy gathered around the table, and lunch was served. Everything looked and smelled so delicious.

Soon Arun's Mummy brought a round chocolate layer cake to the table with ten lit candles on it. As she placed the cake in front of Arun, everyone sang happy birthday. Arun's eyes glistened in delight and with just one breath he blew all the candles out.

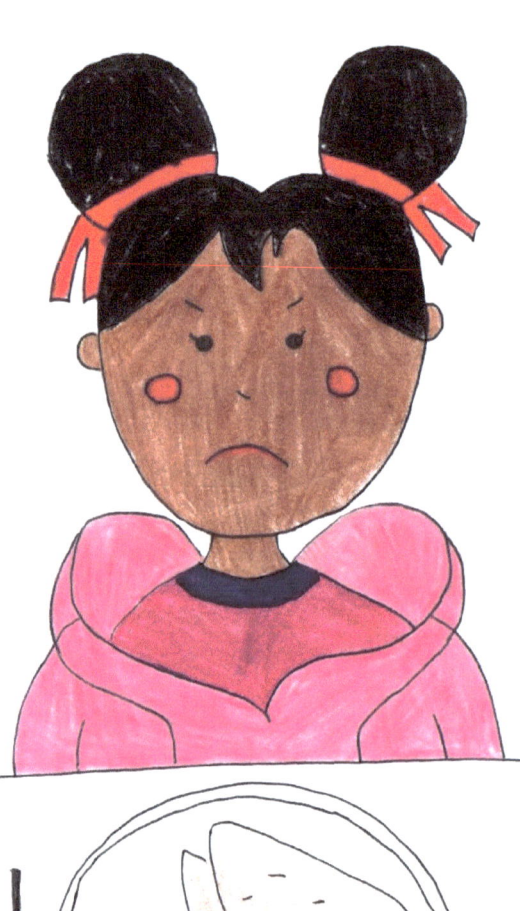

"I'll cut this cake and serve it with the rest of the dessert after dinner, "said Arun's Mummy.

Once everyone began eating, six-year-old Neha wanted to know what her big brother, Arun, had wished for.

"It's a secret, silly! You're not supposed to ask. If I tell you, then my wish won't come true! "Arun replied to his little sister sternly.

Neha just pouted and continued to break her naan. Andy was pretty comfortable eating with his hands just like the rest of Arun's family.

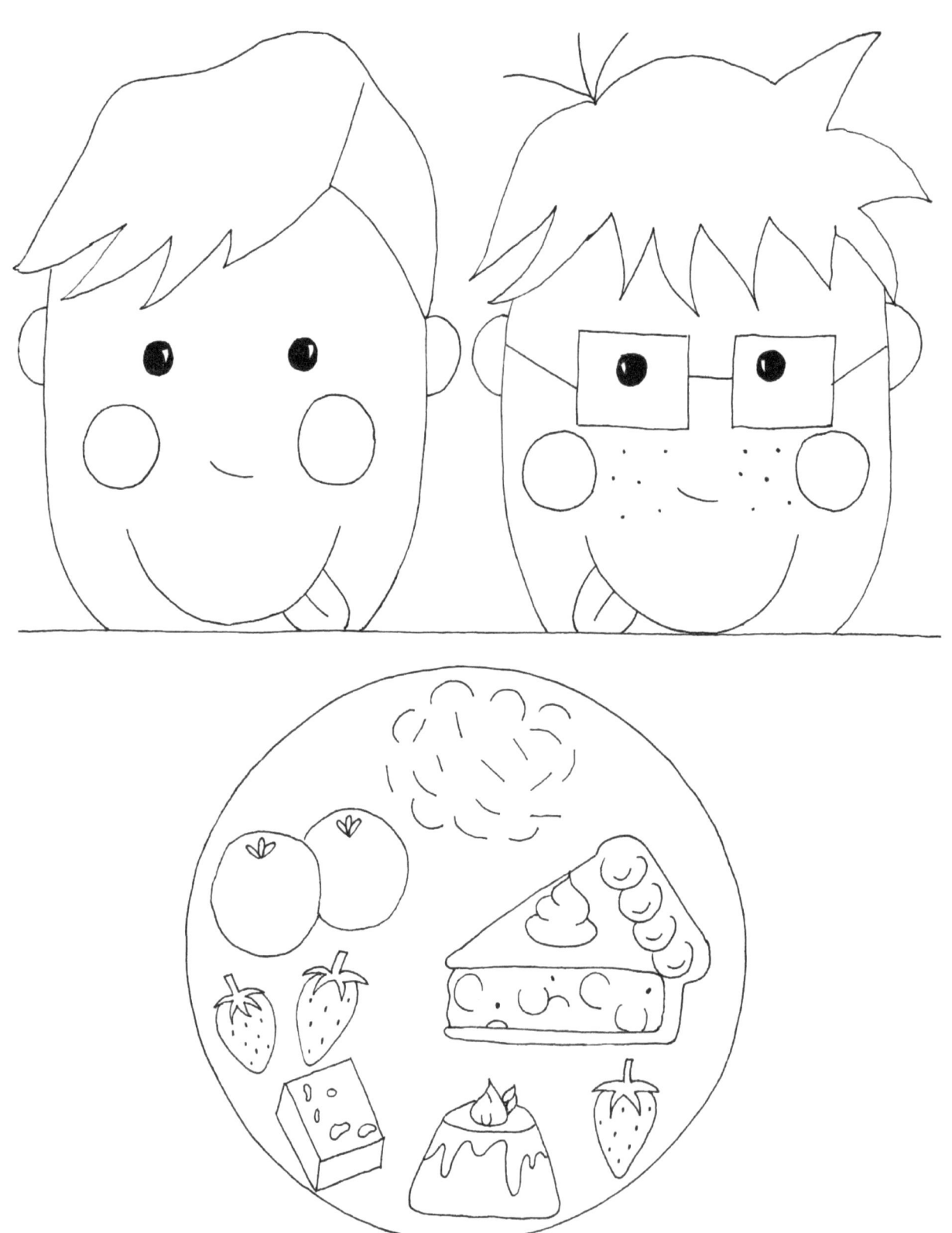

Andy would often go to Arun's house so he became familiar with some of the Indian traditions. The Indian food was spicy, but nothing Andy couldn't handle.

Just as lunch was over, Arun's Mummy brought out the cake slices, gulab jamun, and carrot halwa. Both Arun and Andy's eyes beamed, as their mouths watered. They both wished they could eat it all.

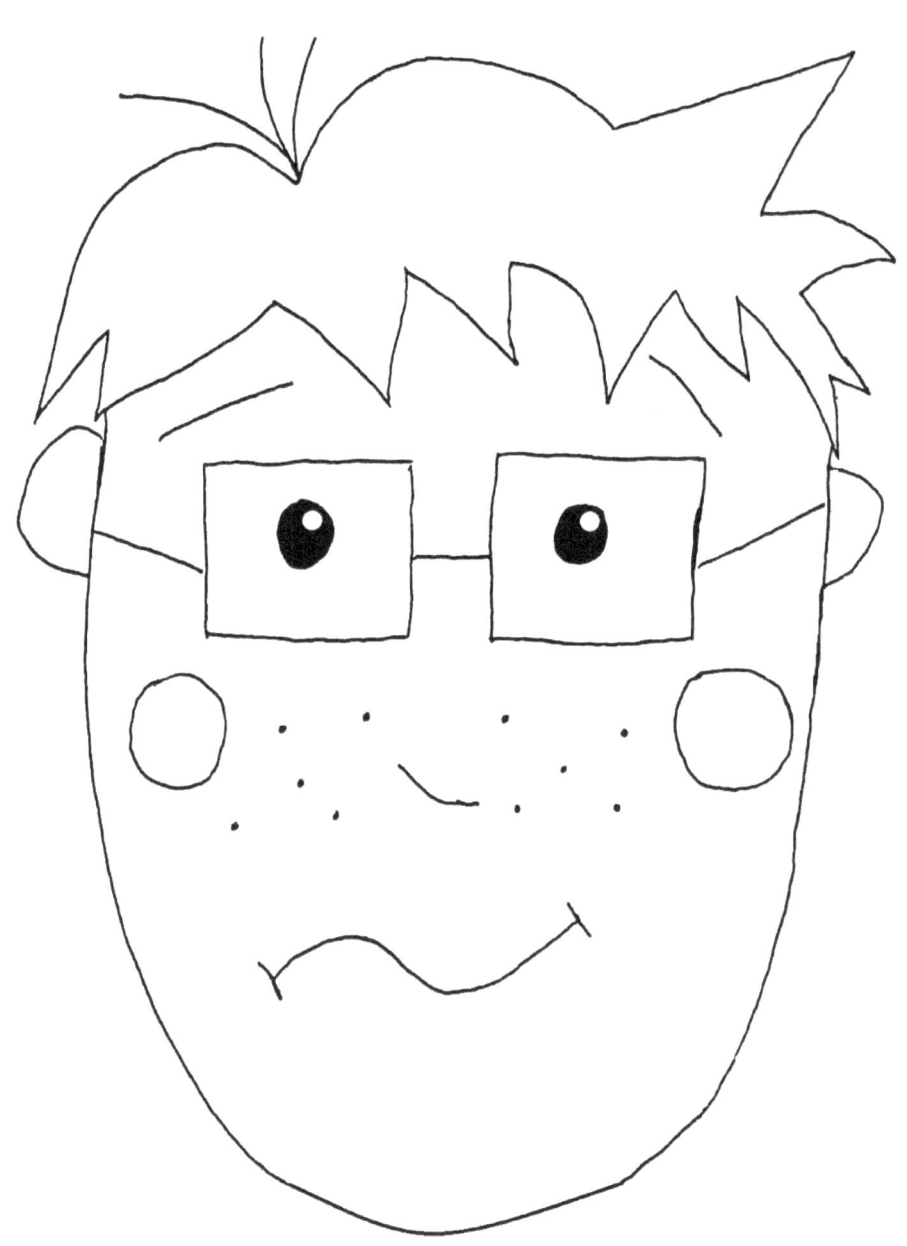

Suddenly Dada asked, "So Andy, do you brush and floss your teeth?"

Andy looked up, quickly swallowed bits of something delicious in his mouth, and blurted,

"Of course! I mean, yes sir, I do."

"How about cleaning your tongue?" Arun's Dada asked.

Andy looked baffled. He shook his head side-to-side slowly, "Uh uh, no sir."

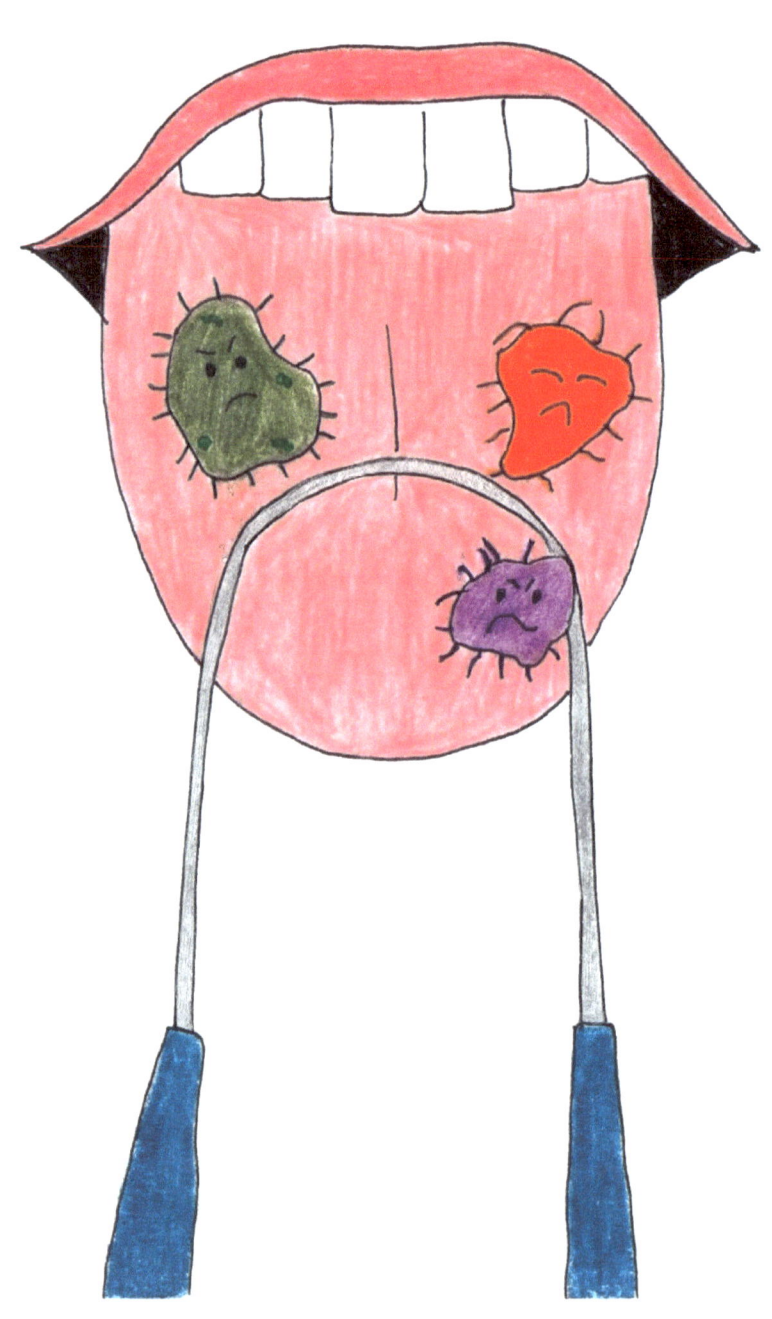

Quietly, everyone turned to pay attention to Dada. "Did you know your tongue has thousands of germs living on it, just like your teeth? Good germs help to digest the food you eat and bad germs on the tongue can cause bad breath, poor digestion, and an unhealthy body. There are parts on the tongue that when kept clean, actually help the organs in our body stay healthy."

All this sounded very interesting to Andy. Dada further added, "Have you noticed how white your tongue gets overnight from eating certain things? All that yucky coating comes from the leftover food that sticks to your tongue if it isn't cleaned."

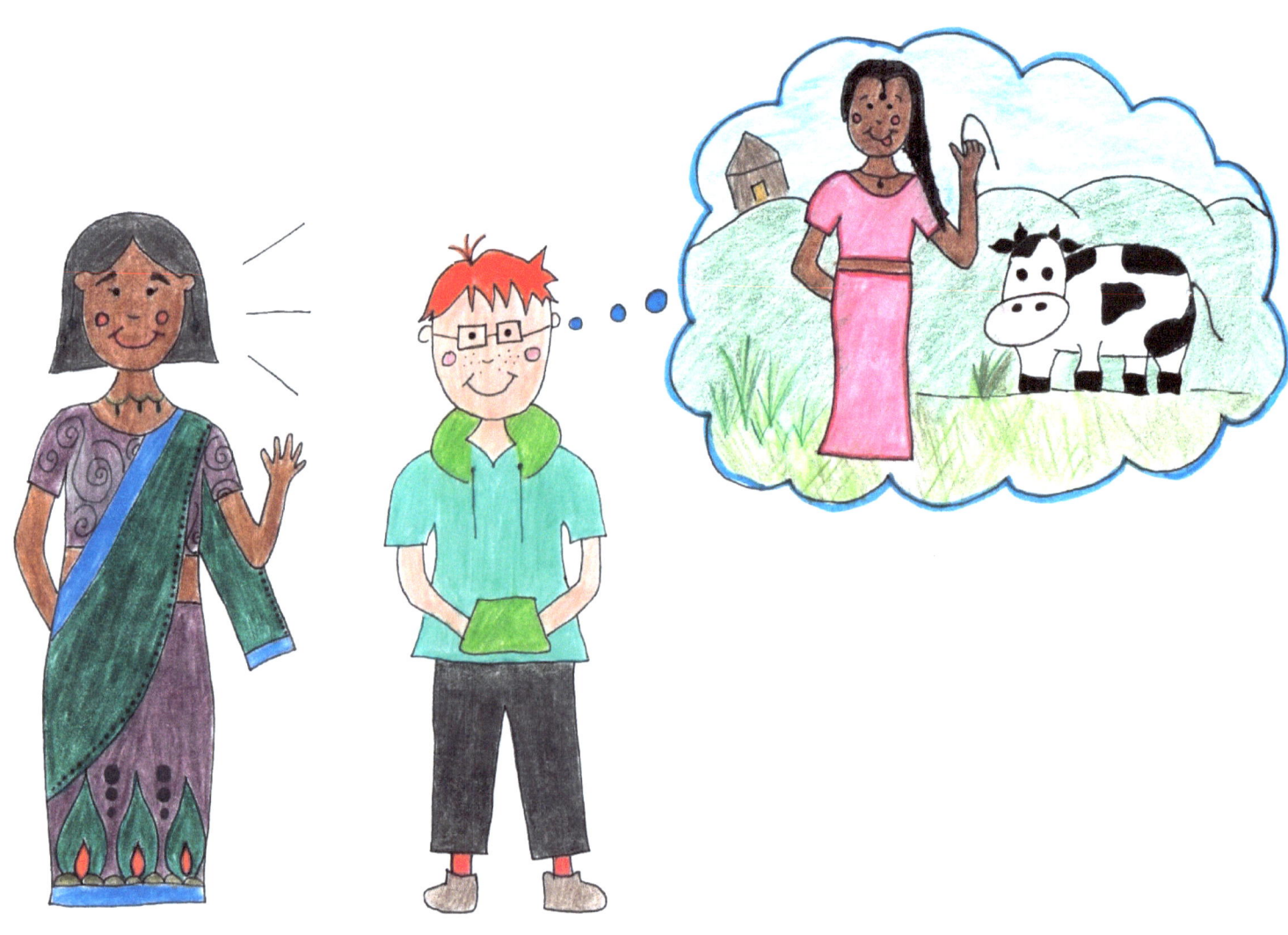

"Yes," Arun's grandma, Dadi, added, "For many, many years, people in India have been cleaning their tongues as part of their brushing routine."

Dadi asked Andy, "Did you know Ayurveda is the traditional system of Indian medicine that helps keep us healthy?"

Andy obviously did not know this. He shook his head, no.

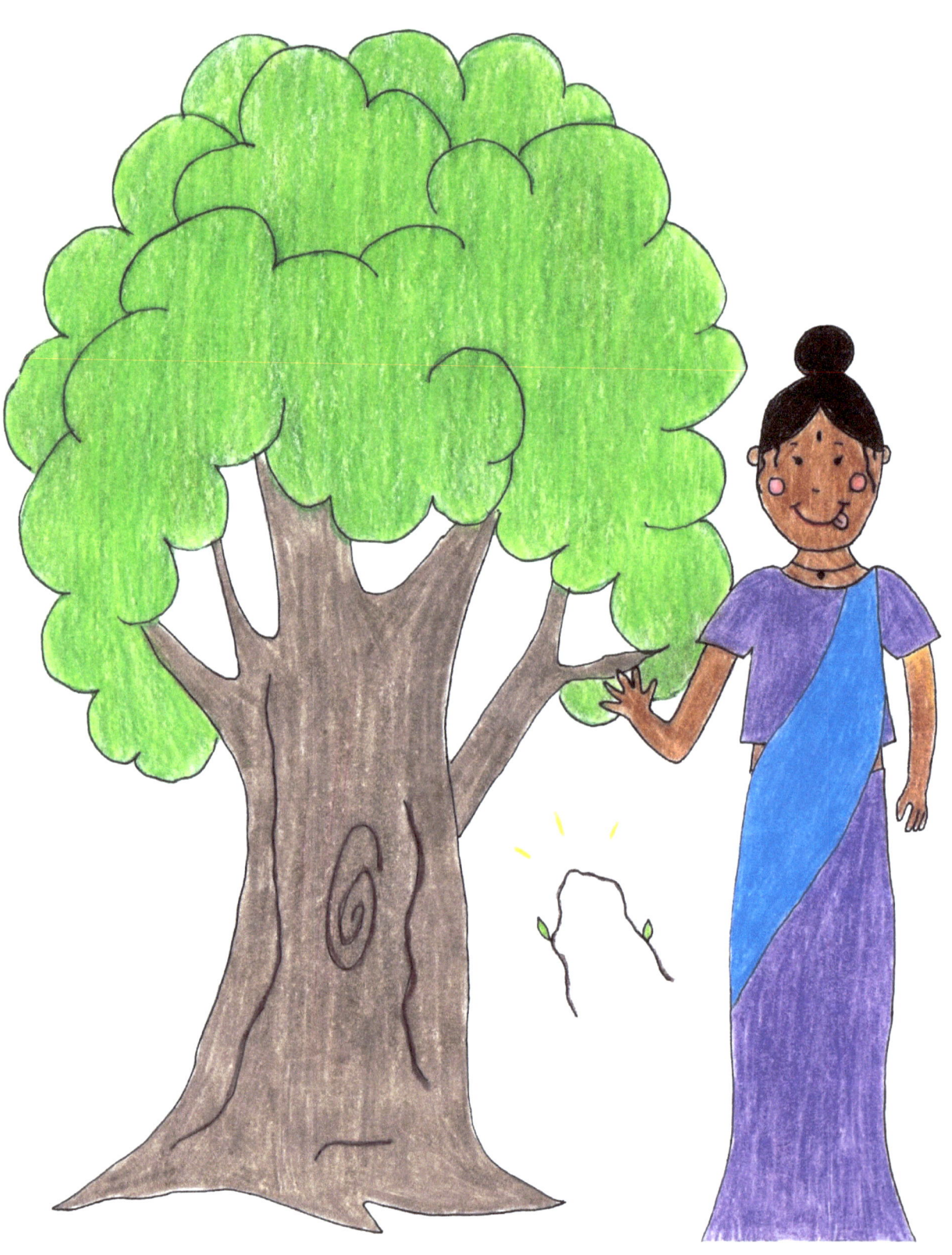

"Some people still use the twigs of certain plants and split them in half to scrape the germs off their tongues. Today you will notice stainless steel "u-shaped" tongue scrapers in most Indian homes," Dadi explained.

Andy smiled as he liked learning new things.

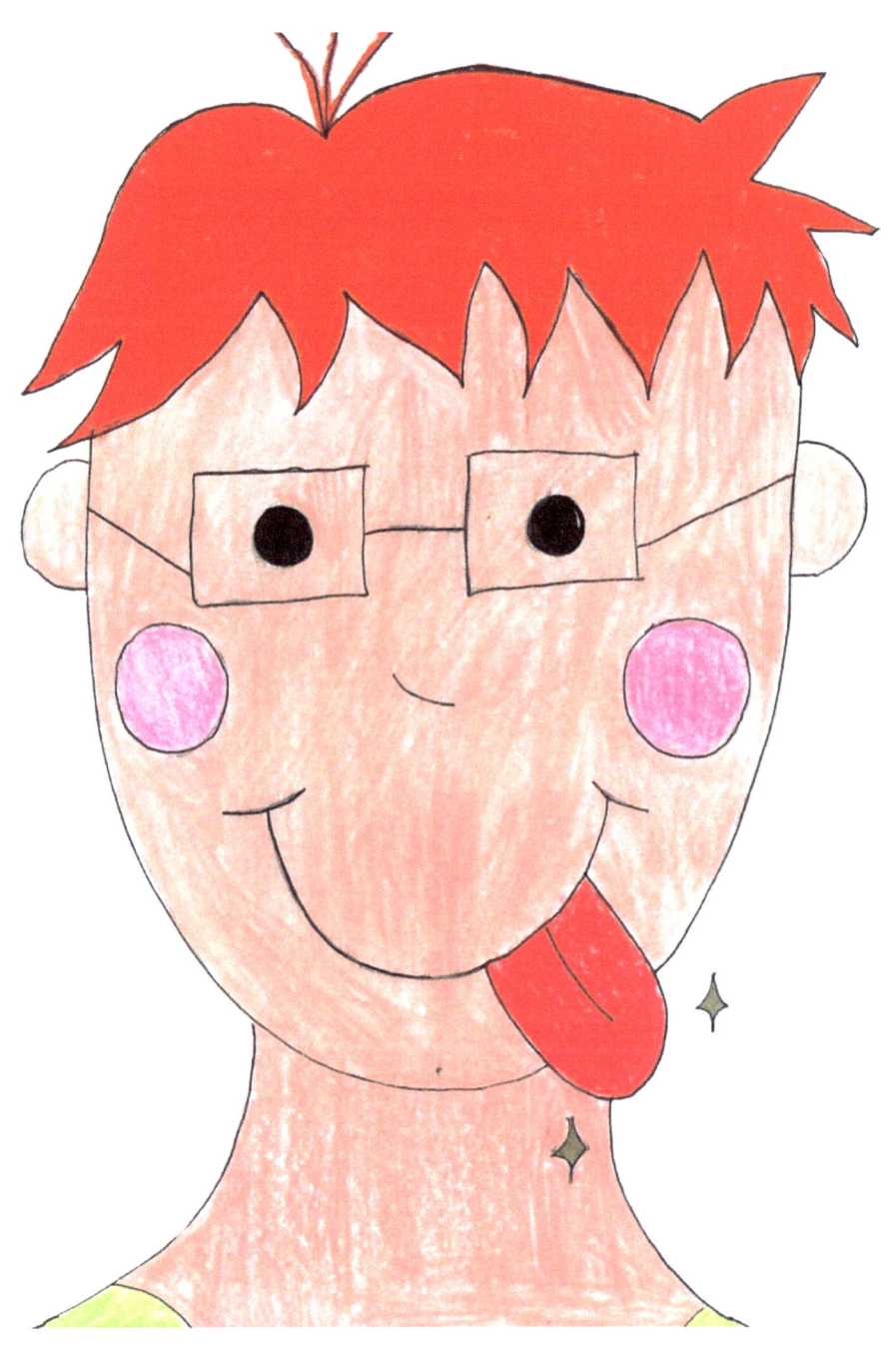

"So, see Andy, scraping your tongue helps to aid in digesting your food and it also gives your tongue a massage at the same time."

Dada continued, "Toothbrushes are meant for cleaning solid teeth surfaces, but on a spongy muscle like the tongue, a metal scraper removes unwanted germs and left-over food particles. More so, tongue cleaning will make you have a fresh clean breath. It's just as important as brushing and flossing."

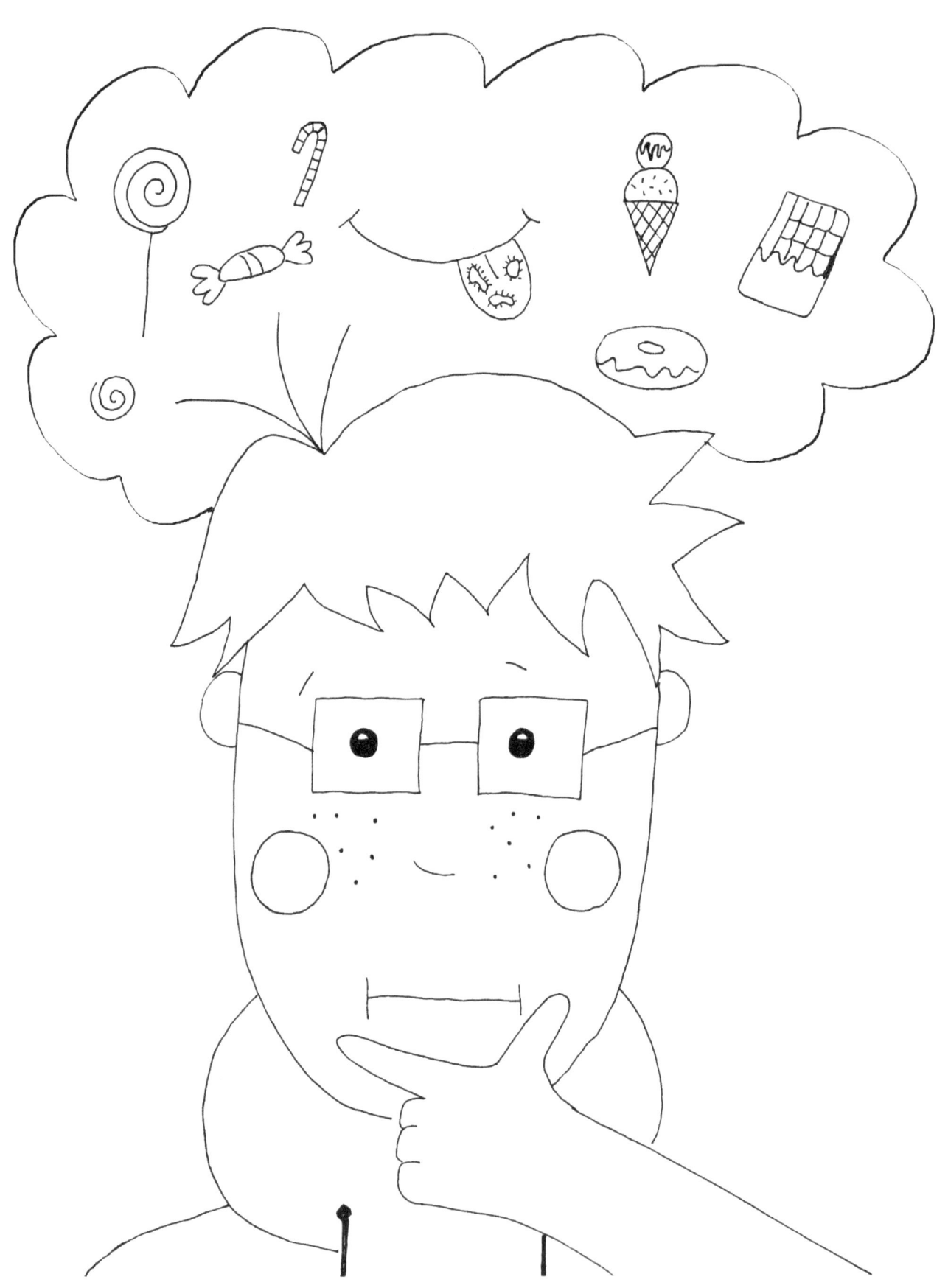

"You will absolutely love it, Andy!"

said Arun.

"Especially every day it will make your mouth feel awake and all the good food will taste even better!"

As Andy was swallowing his dessert, he began thinking about how all the sugars from the food were going to make his tongue white.

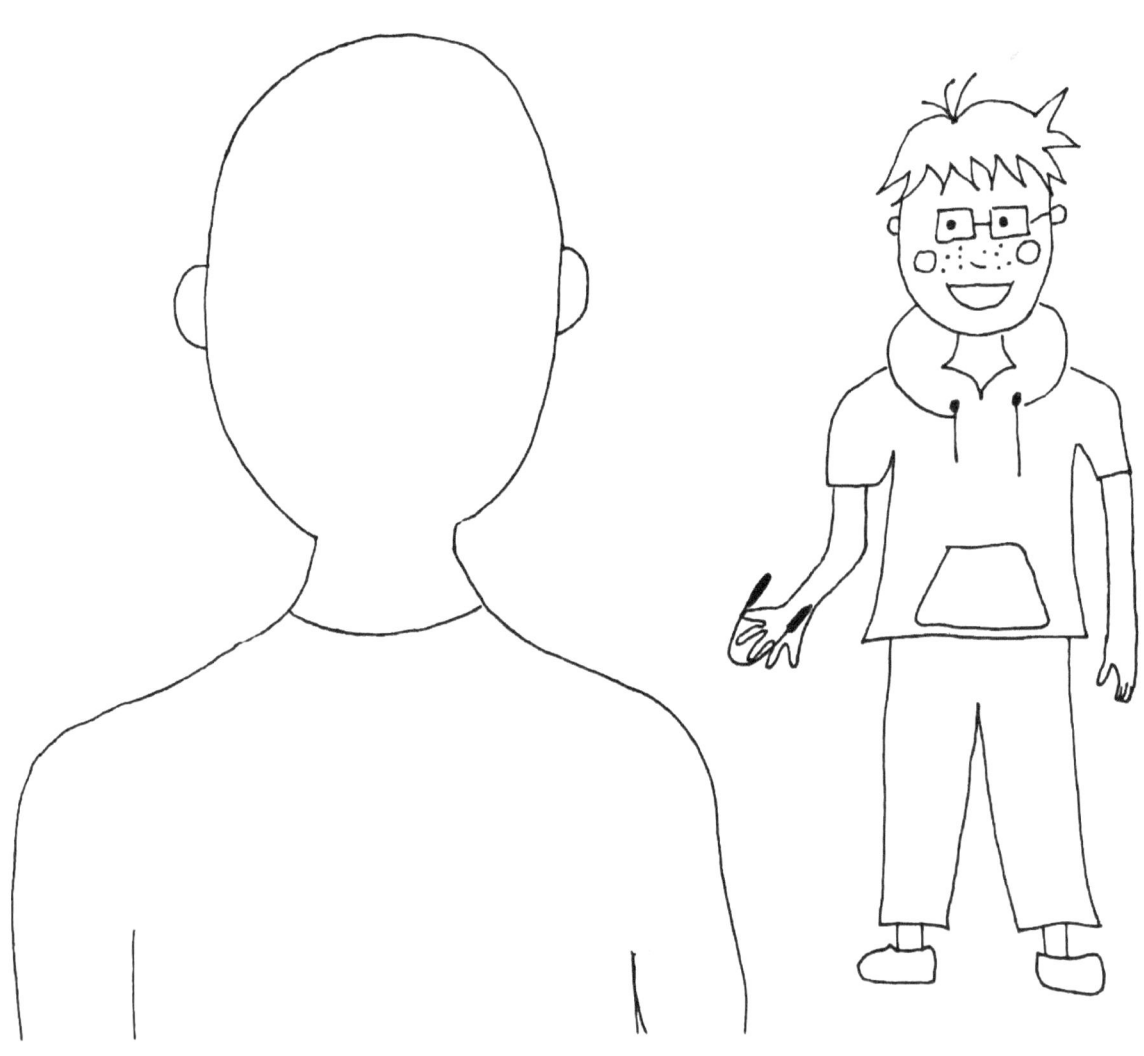

Just then Papa, Arun's dad, handed Andy a brand-new metal tongue scraper.

"Here you go, Andy, give it a try and see what you think."

It was one of the best party favors Andy had ever received.

"I will definitely use it, sir!"

Andy replied excitedly.

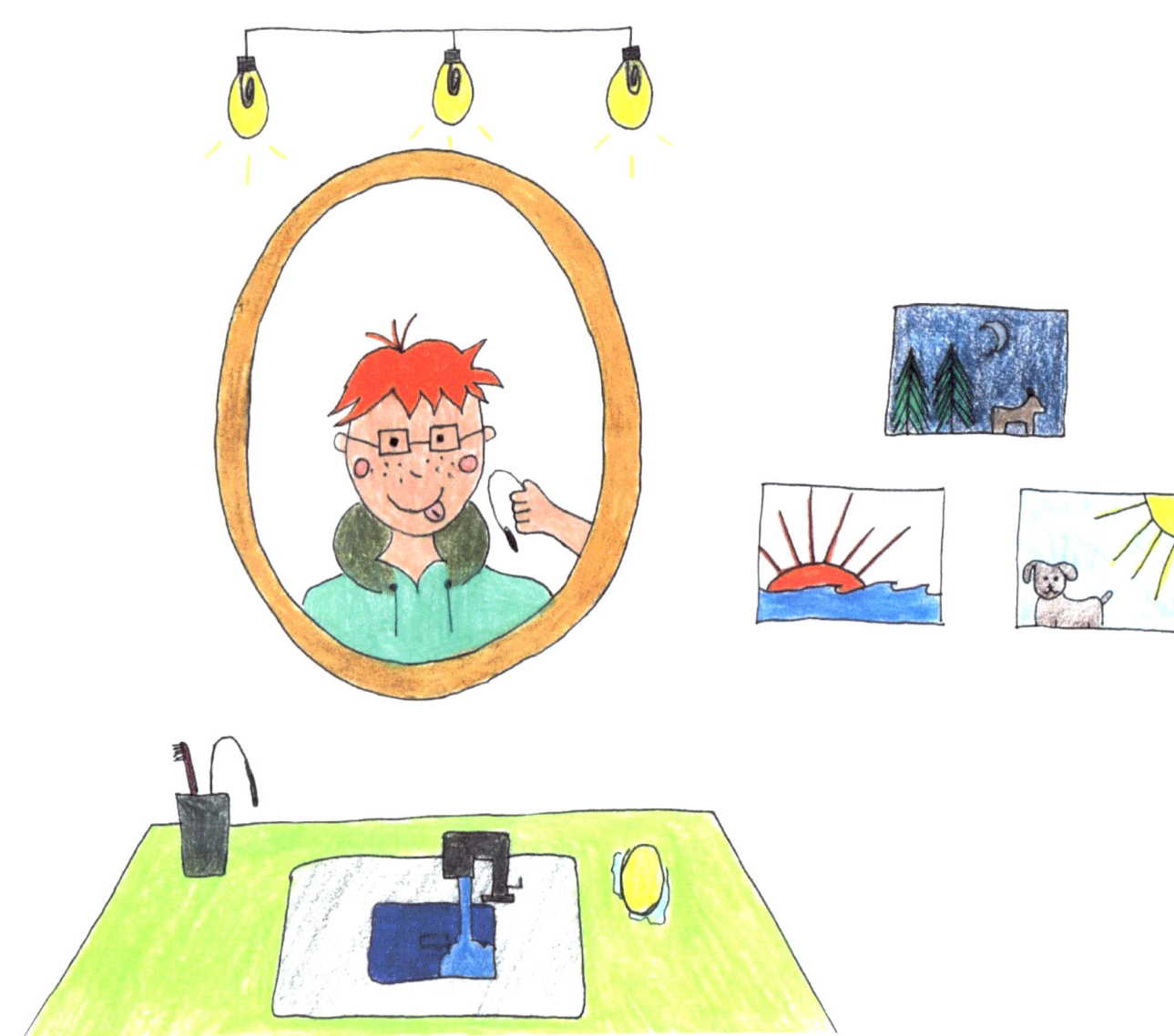

After saying goodbye and thanking Arun and his family for the tasty meal, Andy rushed back home. He couldn't wait to try his new, shiny tongue scraper.

He went straight into the bathroom, brushed his teeth, scraped his tongue and then stuck his tongue out.

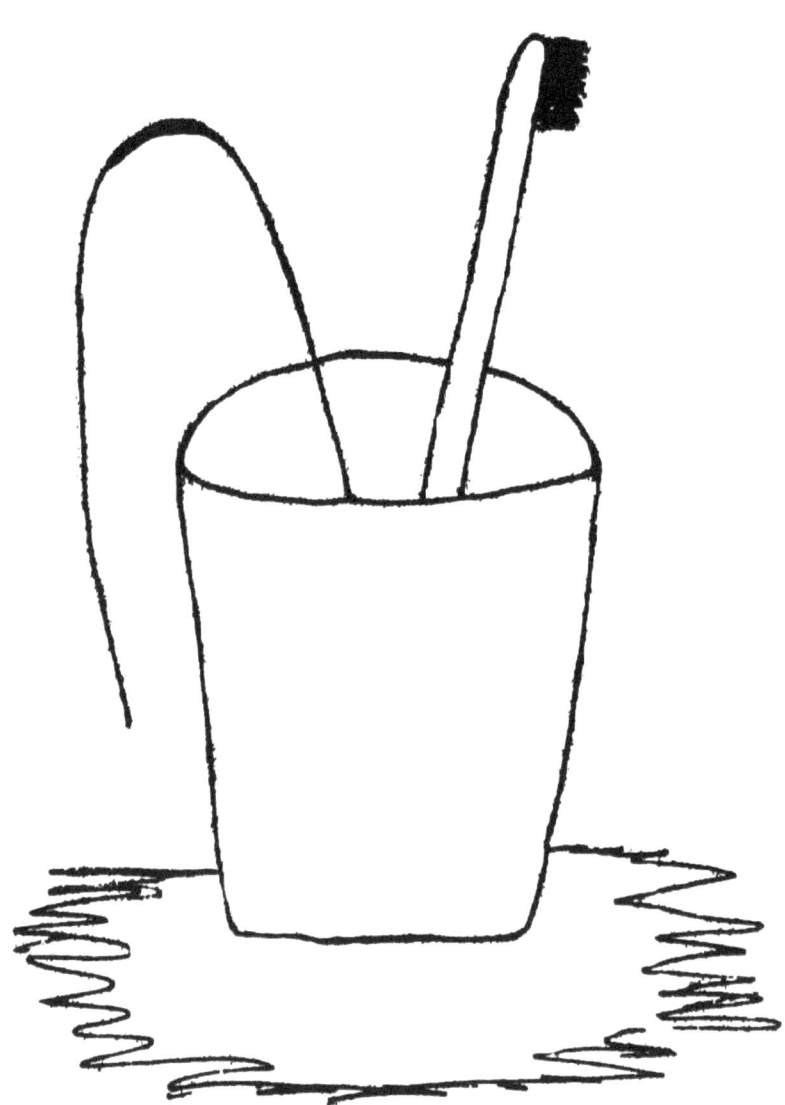

"Oh boy!" Andy exclaimed as he looked in the mirror and saw no more white stuff on his tongue.

Andy's whole mouth felt clean and his breath felt fresh, too! Dada was right.

"I bet my Mom and Dad will not be able to guess what I learned today at Arun's place.

I promise to use my tongue scraper every day, and teach everyone around me the importance of cleaning their tongues." said Andy. From then on Andy kept his promise.

THE END

Scrape That Tongue

By Keyan Patel

Your tongue is filled with a lot of germs

Little critters that move like worms,

Your tongue is stained by white gunk after you eat

A bunch of sticky particles make up this sheet,

So please take care of your tongue,

It doesn't matter whether you're old or young,

Remember to brush, floss, and scrape that tongue!

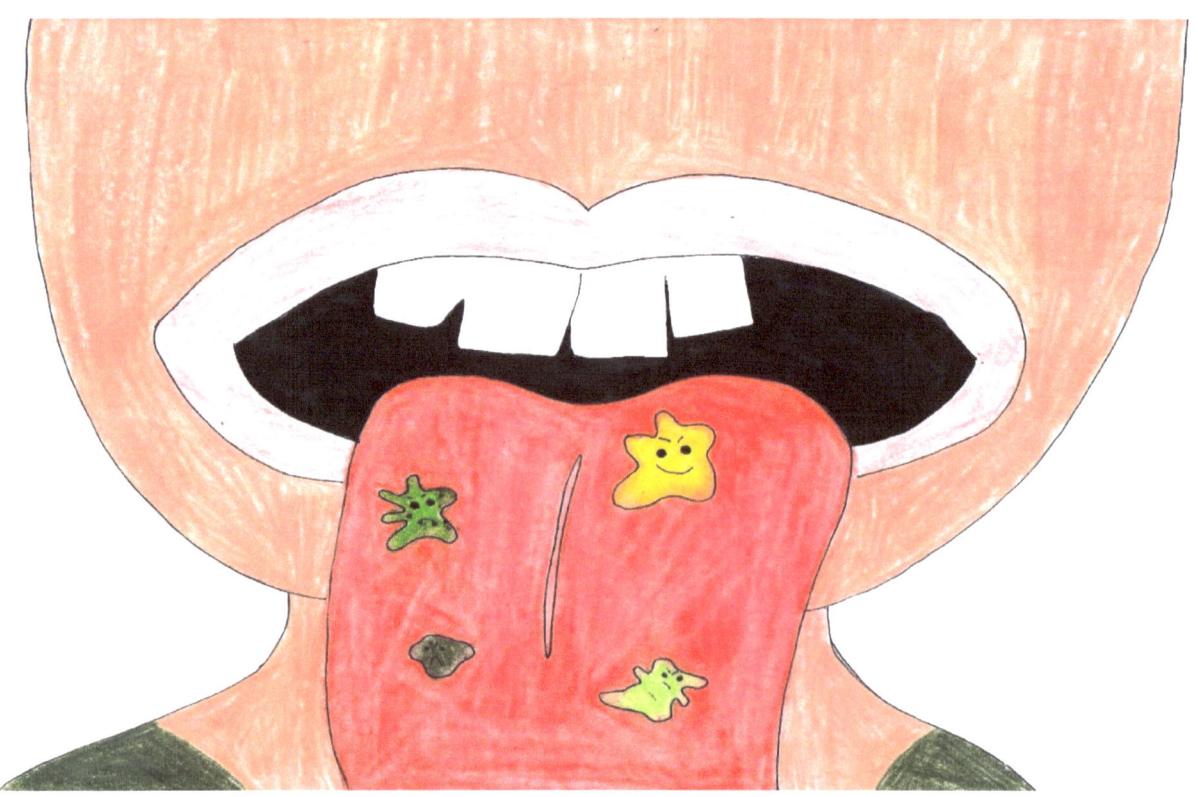

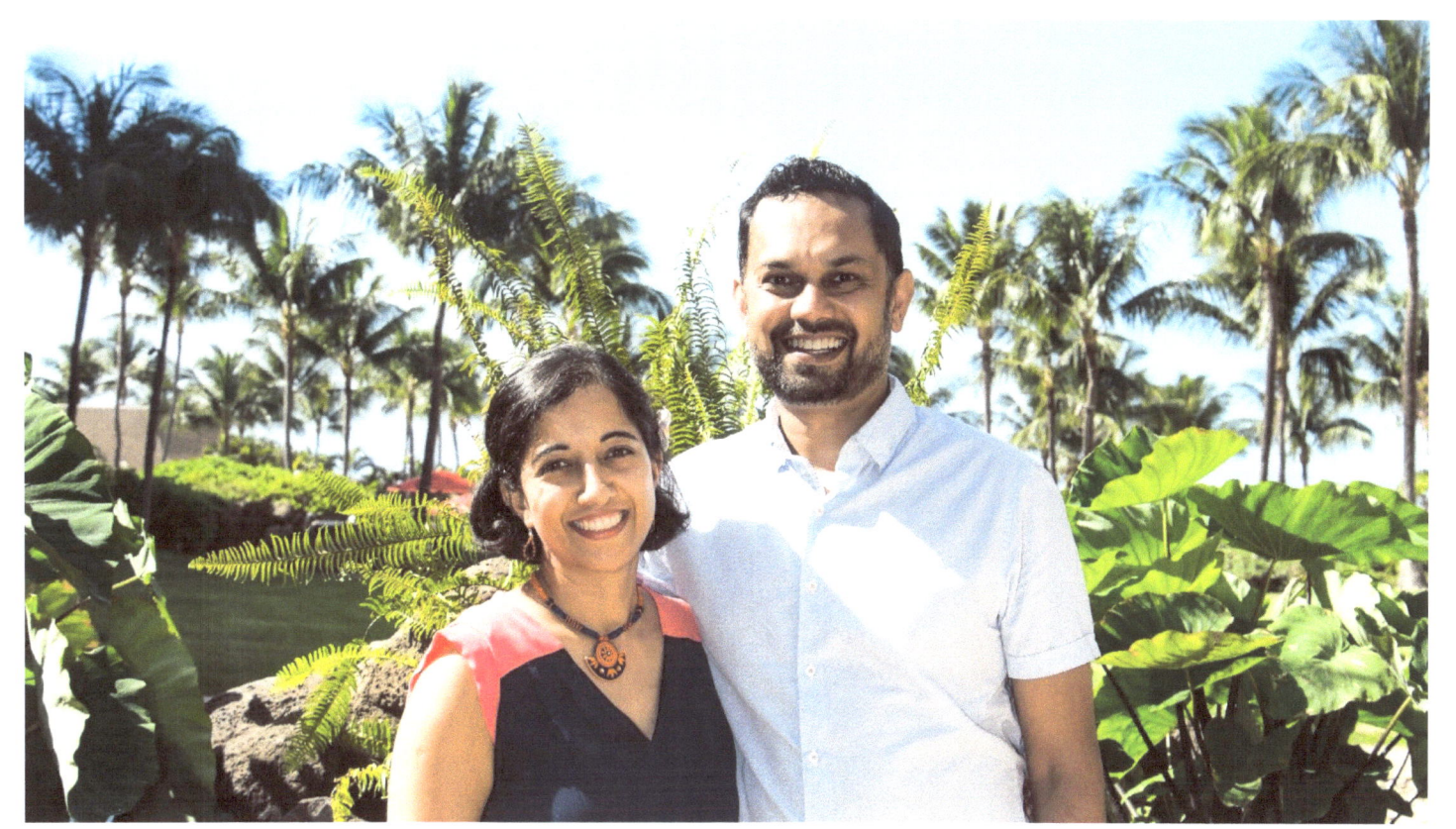

Sangita Patel

Author

Sangita Patel is an Indian girl who was born and raised in Africa. She moved to the USA at the age of 16. She now lives on the beautiful Central Coast of California. She worked with children as a dental assistant for many years. Sangita loves to spend time with her family, cook and travel.

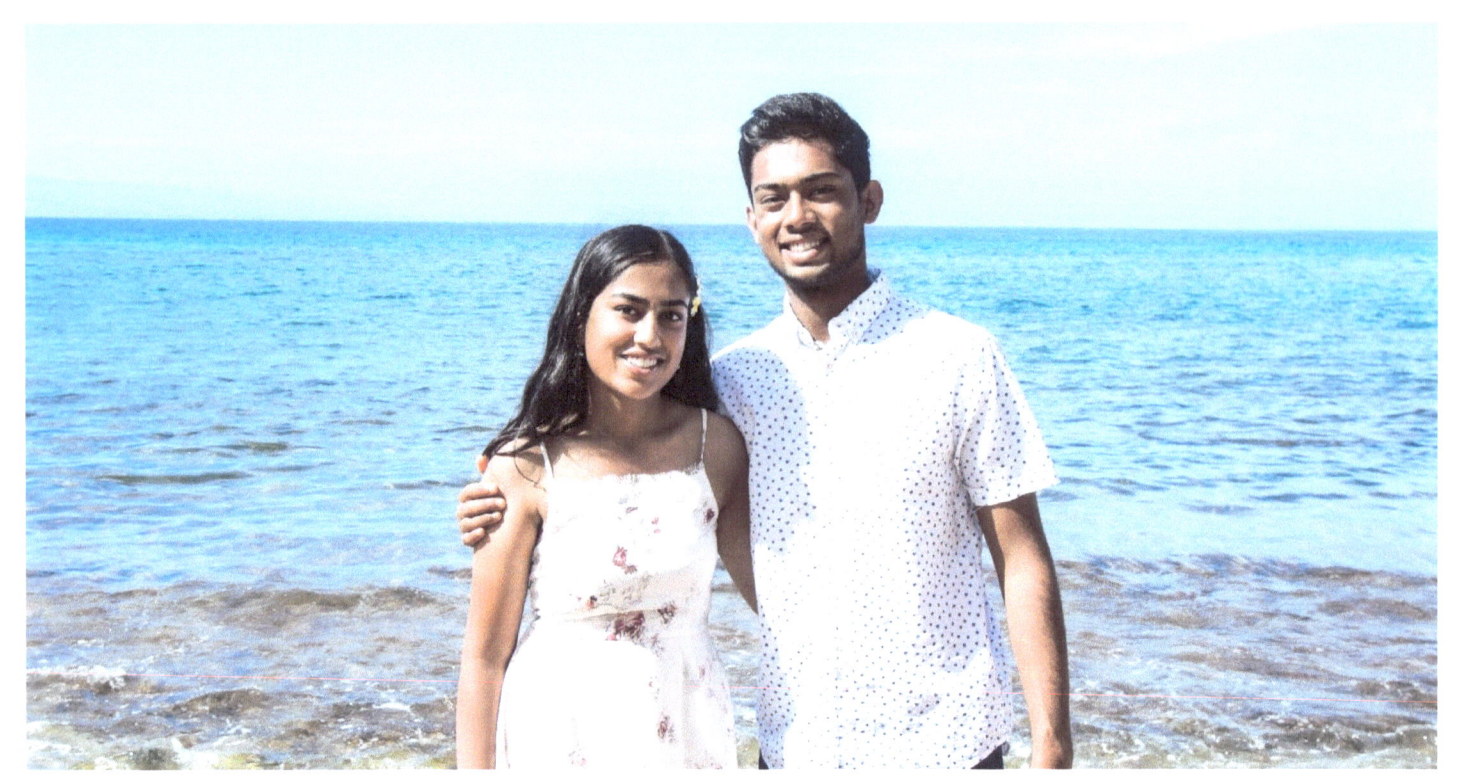

Siona Patel

Illustrator

Siona Patel, is the author's daughter, a beautiful young lady who loves painting, traveling and reading.

Keyan Patel

Poet

Keyan Patel is the author's son, a tall, handsome young man who enjoys the outdoors and learning new things every day.

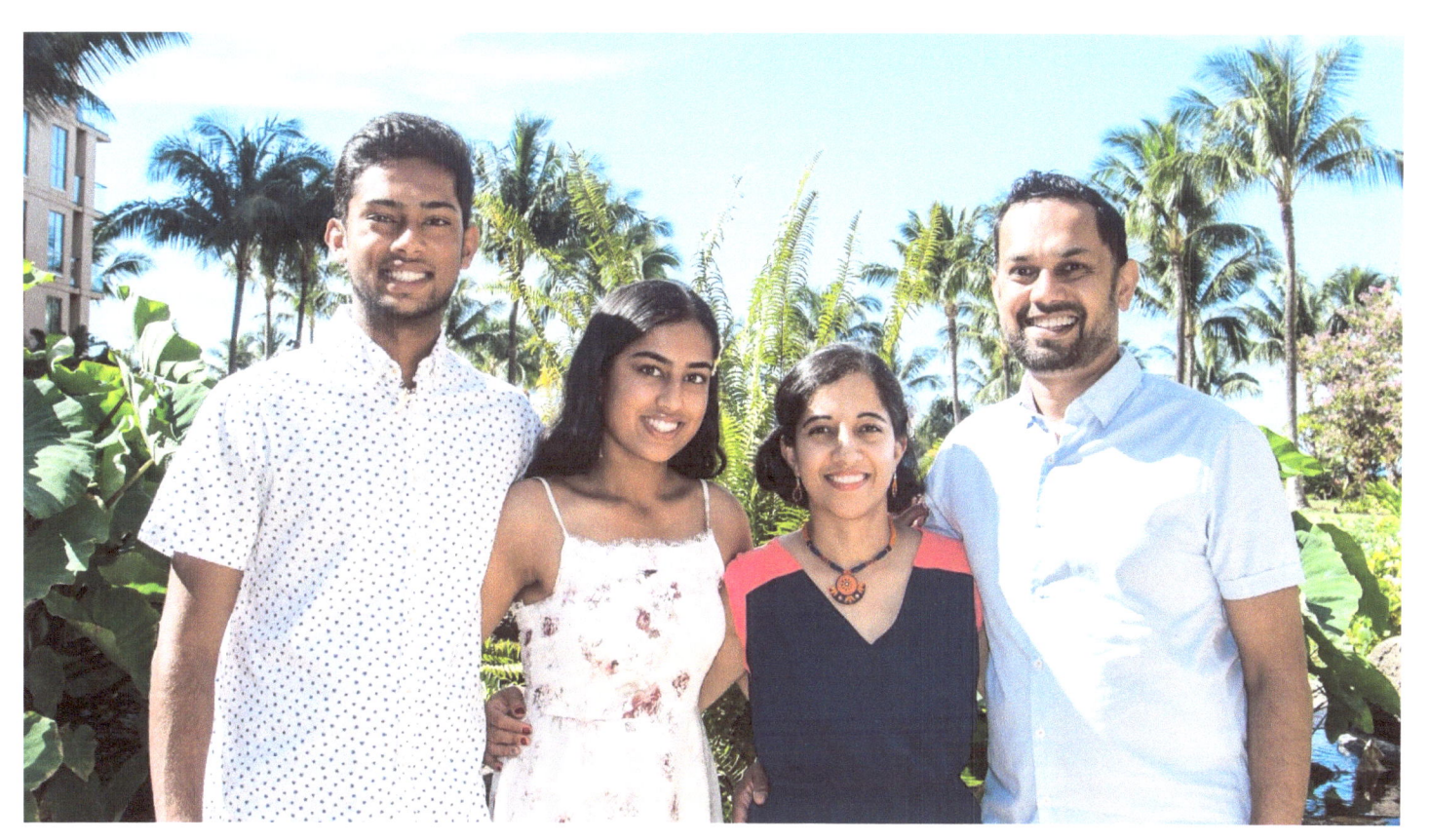

Dr. Perry Patel

Contributor

Dr. Perry Patel, is Sangita's husband. He is a well-known dentist in the Five Cities area of Pismo Beach, CA. He loves his job, and his family.

MY TONGUE NEEDS CLEANING, TOO!

Writing and Drawing Prompts:

1. What do you think Arun's big birthday gift was? Draw an illustration of a gift you think he would like.

2. Make a birthday card for your best friend and be sure to write a special message.

3. Have you ever eaten Indian food? Describe what it tasted like and felt like to you? What was your favorite dish? Draw a picture of what you ate.

4. How would you keep your mouth clean every day? What foods help to keep your teeth strong and your body healthy?

5. Draw objects you use every day to have a clean mouth.

6. Describe the people in your family and what traditions you celebrate. List one thing you learned from your grandparents.

www.ingramcontent.com/pod-product-compliance
Lightning Source LLC
Chambersburg PA
CBHW051216220526
45473CB00003B/1050